FRONTIERS
The Journey of Two Surgeons Through Stroke

Dr. Siva Murugappan M.D, FRCS(C)
Dr. Prema Samy M.D, FRCS(C)

◆ **FriesenPress**

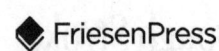

One Printers Way
Altona, MB R0G 0B0
Canada

www.friesenpress.com

Copyright © 2023 by Dr. Siva Murugappan and Dr. Prema Samy
First Edition — 2023

Audrey Ansell/Amy Wilcox - Ghost Writers

All rights reserved.

No part of this publication may be reproduced in any form, or by any means, electronic or mechanical, including photocopying, recording, or any information browsing, storage, or retrieval system, without permission in writing from FriesenPress.

ISBN
978-1-03-917644-7 (Hardcover)
978-1-03-917643-0 (Paperback)
978-1-03-917645-4 (eBook)

1. BIOGRAPHY & AUTOBIOGRAPHY, PERSONAL MEMOIRS

Distributed to the trade by The Ingram Book Company

I dedicate this book to my mother,
Kamala Murugappan

Foreword

Dr. Prema Samy (wife of Dr. Siva Murugappan)

The idea for this book was conceived when Siva was in the early days of recovery in the stroke unit. I found a few memoirs in the small library in the rehabilitation ward, of people who have survived strokes. I learnt a lot about the struggles of families, but as Siva's journey evolved, I felt that maybe his was a story worth telling, as he has very specialized skills. The multitude of emotions, struggles, and roadblocks he overcame may help and inspire another person who is on a similar journey. Even if only one person is inspired, this book will have been worth writing.

Acknowledgements

Dr. Siva Murugappan

I am where I am today because of the grace of God, who spared my life and seasoned it with many souls, for whom I am grateful.

To my wife, Prema, my best friend, my rock, who was always there to assist, guide, support, and encourage me.

To my children, Arjun and Geetha, who went through this journey with me and were loving and patient.

To my mother, always my pillar of strength. To my family in Malaysia and India, who prayed for my recovery and whose love and affection I know I always have.

To the Chatham-Kent Health Alliance: the physicians who cared for me, the nurses on the rehab floor, the therapists who worked with me, and the Alliance, for its much-appreciated support. I am proud to say that my complete recovery and rehabilitation happened here. I continue to work here with gratitude.

To the many nurses who supported me, especially Shauna. To colleagues who encouraged me. To my buddies, Kasi, Ramesh, and Balaji.

To Sandi, my personal trainer. Thank you for your constant encouragement and tough love. I would also like to make special mention of David Menor, my personal support worker, who is no longer with us. Thank you so much, David. I will never forget the care that you provided me.

I would also like to thank Nilda, Elaine, Charlotte, Anita, and Tabitha.

I am grateful to Audrey, who was our ghostwriter and good friend. Talking about my emotions and struggles with you for the book was therapeutic for me. Thank you to Amy, my daughter-in-law, who helped finish this book and made it a reality.

Last, but most important, is my golden retriever, Benji, my constant companion and angel. I love you forever.

Contents

Prologue 1
Falling off the Precipice, One Stroke at a Time 3
September 27, 2017—The Day Everything Changed 7
Discharge 13
Way Back When 19
Scaling Great Heights to a Stroke 23
Get Back to Where You Once Belonged 27
Prema as Sherpa 33
Patience, Patients, Patience, Patients 37
Children 39
Fit to Go Back 43
Waiting Game 49
Now What? 53
Back to the Grind 55
Fair Is Fair, Purpose of Purpose 57
The Mechanics of Breaching a Frontier 61
Perspectives—Different Views of the Same Thing 65
Wherever He Goes, Ego Goes Too 69
Regrouping for the Final Ascent 73
The Battle Within 75
Global Pandemic 77
Epilogue 79
Thoughts on the Regulatory and Life Expedition 85
Abbreviations used in book 90
Resources—Signs of Stroke 91
Local Chatham-Kent Protocol for Stroke 93

Do not learn how to react, learn how to respond.
—Buddha

Prologue

A frontier is an area beyond a boundary. I have lived my life in this space, always overcoming hurdles and pushing forward, always looking to the horizon for what's coming next. Predicting, speculating, adapting, reacting. I have diagnosed, repaired, and consoled many people in my clinic, in the operating room, and on the ward. My brain has been wired to focus for hours through complex surgeries while managing staff and encouraging junior doctors. Throughout my journey of becoming a surgeon, I have felt confident in the decisions and actions that I have chosen to make. I have always known my life to be under my control, and now it is not. I had a right brain ischemic stroke.

"We don't know. We don't know. We don't know."

Every stroke is different, so there is no simple answer to give someone about how they will recover, repair, reboot, or restore. What a damning prognosis for a surgeon. Now, I am a stroke survivor.

It was never planned this way, of course, but I am confident that my entire life has prepared me for this new space. What if I can recover better than anyone else? I want to diagnose, explore, and suture again. I want to run. The clinicians, my own colleagues, said that it might not be possible. I have never run before, so why start now? I can see the skepticism surrounding me. No one can understand that I am not interested in just running. I want to jump hurdles too, to break through to new frontiers again.

The real stroke, I am coming to see, has been one of luck, good fortune, and destiny. Among this trifecta, I consider trying to mask the tell-tale limp, and I strive to overcome the involuntarily raised left arm. These are the lasting souvenirs from the early hours of my stroke journey. But now, I am even more complex and refined; my senses and sensitivities are heightened. I am made from pressures and forces; the fissures let the light in.

I am Siva. This story is my personal destiny.

This is my frontier.

Falling off the Precipice, One Stroke at a Time

Siva

Work and patients came first, and my needs and those of my family came second. Now, with the benefit of hindsight, what a ridiculously short-sighted prioritization that was. My days as a high-performing general surgeon were very different to those of most other general surgeons in my peer group. I saw more patients and worked longer hours than anyone else. When it came to work, "no" was never a part of my vocabulary. Consequently, I had great performance statistics with which to relish and often regale people. Then, out of the blue, I became something of a statistic myself.

September 27, 2017, was no different from any other day, not for me, anyway. I was powering through a particularly lengthy session with a very large polyp I was trying to remove endoscopically to finish the day in the endoscopy suite. As usual, there had been no time for breaks, no time for a bite to eat or a sip to drink. This was, however, no big deal, as I was trained to power through old-school style.

Waiting on the third floor for the elevator, I received a call from the emergency room (ER). A patient, a sex worker who had been dealt a tough hand in life, had been admitted to the hospital with a bad abscess on her leg. As I momentarily conjured up an image of her, I was cast back to a vagrant in India whom I had once saved from certain death. Someone else who needed help. I briefly considered whether to hit the "G" button in the elevator, head down to the ground floor and home to rest and eat. In other words, to put my needs first and then come back to take care of the patient. Instead, I entered the elevator and pressed the button for the fourth floor.

I started the procedure to incise the abscess bedside on the ward floor. Then something in my head shifted. The grip in my left hand went, and my legs buckled. Catching the surgical instruments tray as I fell, the noise of it crashing to the floor was almighty and brought nurses running from all corners. They sat me in a chair, and one of the nurses noticed the droopy muscles in my face. Stroke. We all knew.

Everyone sprang into action and a stretcher soon arrived for me. I sat on it without any assistance. Lying back, I was waving my arms and moving my legs in any way possible to show them that I was okay. I wanted to be stronger than this.

Within ten minutes, I was in the emergency department, and that's when the fog soon descended. I was aware of what was happening to me. A computerized tomography (CT) scan was ordered, and I felt the heat surge through me, immediately recognizing it as the contrast flowed through my veins.

A neurologist from London, Ontario, read the results of the CT scan remotely, diagnosing an ischemic stroke in my right brain and indicating that there was no need for a thrombectomy. I was started on tissue plasminogen activator (tPA), a clot-busting drug. Within minutes, I was moving my arms and legs, especially my left side which was weak earlier. I kept thinking to myself, This is amazing, *I* am amazing— I'm going to beat a stroke.

Then my wife, Prema, arrived in the emergency department, and reality struck. I knew this from the look on her face. While I felt lively, I realized that was not how things looked through her eyes. There I was, in a bed, in the ER, in the hospital where we both worked. There I lay, surrounded by our colleagues, with a stroke, with my ability to control my movements fading. That's when my tears came freely and without any inhibition. This freedom of expression is apparently a gift to stroke patients— emotions run high. My tears were not just for me; right then, they were for the burden I believed I would become. They were for work and surgeries that would be lost and for the unknown of what was to come.

I was moved to the intensive care unit (ICU) after tPA in the ER, and the impact my little stroke had was palpable. My neurological status was under constant watch; I was bedridden and could not move. This close monitoring was to be alert for another stroke, which can, after tPA, sometimes cause brain bleed. After three days, I was moved to the stroke recovery unit.

After ten days of lying in bed, I was mobilized. A wheelchair became my new mode of transport. I tried my best to remain upbeat and refused to allow the paralysis of my left side to rule me. I tried to use the washroom one night alone. I fell and stayed there, lying in my own urine, until someone came along and sat me upright like a skittle at the bowling alley. Strike.

The news of my stroke spread throughout the entire hospital. What a wake-up call for everyone who was pushing themselves to their frontiers and beyond. No one could quite believe it had happened to one of their own. People lined up outside my door to see me—the nurses wanted to shoo them away, but I accepted that people wanted to see me, to see how bad I looked. They were paying their respects to the end of a career.

Cognitive tests were administered, and I didn't perform well. This was probably due to brain edema or swelling from the stroke. The prognosis and rumours were that Siva was finished.

September 27, 2017—The Day Everything Changed

Prema

My husband is a man accustomed to being in control—he is a surgeon. So, receiving a phone call to tell me that Siva was in the emergency room completely rocked my world.

It was the usual Wednesday afternoon in my office. I had seen the typical array of patients for the usual consults that an ear, nose, and throat (ENT) specialist sees. As I was finishing my dictation, a fellow doctor called my phone, asking where I was. I replied that I was still plugging away at the office. There was a momentary pause, and then I heard, "We have Siva here. He had a stroke."

I can't quite describe the feeling I had in my body when I heard those words. The bottom just instantly fell out of my world. Something in my body shifted, and my legs buckled. I dropped everything and ran to Charlotte, my secretary, crying. The five-minute drive to the ER felt endless.

Imaginings of what had happened and *why* galloped through my mind as I raced to the hospital.

When I saw him on a stretcher, my legs buckled again because it was not the Siva who I woke up to that morning. It was not the same husband to whom I said goodbye as we both rushed out the door to work. The Siva who lay in front of me was diminished, depleted, and scared; it was someone who resembled him, an imposter in familiar surroundings. When he saw me, he was crying and looked utterly horrified. The left side of his face was slack. I met the neurologist and he quickly explained that a trip to London for endovascular embolectomy was needed. As it transpired, the radiologist in the large stroke centre closest to us had read Siva's scan and saw no embolus, so the decision was made in the ER to tPA him.

After tPA in the ER, Siva was admitted to the intensive care unit. This was to monitor as there was still a high risk for another stroke or brain bleed from using the tPA. I sat by his bedside as he slept, and my mind raced. Do we need a caregiver? What will happen to his huge practice? Will we have to fire our office administrative staff whom we employ? What will the children do? Are our finances okay? Will he recover? I struggled to calm my mind of so many questions and unknowns, which, although they were not the current priority, needed to be resolved quickly. Later, we hired a locum to take over Siva's practice. Finally, reaching that decision quieted my mind momentarily.

After three days, Siva was moved from the ICU to the acute stroke unit. We were transients in the hospital, moving from department to department. We saw a different perspective of the hospital and had the opportunity to experience all aspects of the care our colleagues offered on a range of wards. The community of physicians was in shock; there were lines of visitors outside Siva's door every day. It was heartening to see that so many people cared, and it helped us both, as we felt very far from home. We immigrated from Malaysia in 2005 and have no family in Canada. Regardless, it was beyond disheartening to be living in that situation.

We were eventually moved once more to a new inpatient rehabilitation floor. We were given the option to transfer Siva to a larger rehabilitation centre in London, Ontario, but we decided to stay in Chatham hospital as I continued to work full time and would not be able to see Siva daily and I feared he would feel isolated. Siva was smiling and calm, and I still marvel at his ability to be so pleasant under such stressful circumstances. Most concerning of all was that incontinence took hold and my ever-powerful husband couldn't control his own bladder. This devastated me, but Siva accepted it as he does everything with the cards that have been dealt to him. Physiotherapy and occupational therapy became a full-time job, and the routines of hospital life became firmly ingrained in our lives. This time, however, we had breached a frontier and were on the other side, experiencing hospital life as patients.

On the eleventh day, it was Thanksgiving. Siva had had a good night and forwent a shower (it made him light-headed in the morning, and he wanted to be fighting-fit for physio) and decided a freshen-up would be just fine for someone doing so little in the way of exercise. The first order of the day was a Tim Horton's coffee from the in-hospital concession. Siva was adamant that he wanted to venture out from his confines to get his own coffee, so I pushed him down in his wheelchair, and the customer in front of us bought Siva his time-honoured single-single coffee: one cream and one sugar. We took the elevator back up to the atrium and sat in harmony, enjoying the beautiful day. We talked about the fact that Siva had had a stroke and not a myocardial infarction. We agreed that we had both been completely blindsided. We considered how our colleagues had been impacted. We recognized that we had a lot to be thankful for.

The Thanksgiving physio session was a good one. Siva could bridge—a weight-bearing exercise that increases muscular strength—and they taught him how to transfer in and out of bed. Such simple things to accomplish are ground-breaking for a stroke patient. Siva was ecstatic. With such hope in the air and the prospect that life could go on, I felt secure enough to leave his side and popped out to the office to catch up on my own patient consultation dictations and paperwork.

Day twelve was not as successful. During the night, Siva had bad left-foot spasms, and despite the nurses' best efforts, only tramadol took away the pain. When I got to him in the morning, he looked and sounded exhausted. His nurse, Angie, and I freshened him up, and I got him his regular coffee. The hot beverage pushed Siva into a deep sleep and left me with thoughts about how much our lives had changed. How was Siva going to be able to perform surgeries again? Would we ever go on another vacation and reminisce in the glory of our travel photos? How we would manage financially continued to occupy my mind. Then I looked at the facts in the cold light of day: we were only twelve days post-stroke. I needed to remind myself to be patient, that it was still early days, and there was nothing more to do other than accept the situation and let Siva sleep.

A family meeting was arranged for day fifteen. The therapists, stroke unit nurse, and home services manager were present all together on a Friday afternoon. Each of them stated their goals for Siva and recounted his recovery so far. The physical aspects I could understand—they were there for all to see. However, when the occupational therapist started talking about low cognitive scores and poor spatial orientation both of which were seen as far below average, it was disheartening to me. I couldn't imagine what Siva felt. We both knew that we had a long road ahead.

At five weeks post-stroke, we had a breakthrough, making November 4, 2017, a momentous day. Siva was able to stand up to pee. Who would have thought that performing such a basic human function could be so significant and instill so much hope?

Weeks six and seven post-stroke were tough. November brought rain, and with that came gloomy thoughts. With so much daily effort required to fulfill simple tasks, Siva stated plainly that he wished he had died. This was one of the most difficult things to hear.

The focus continued to be mainly on restoring more of Siva's basic functions, such as walking and moving. Siva's control of his upper limbs was not good, and when I saw this daily struggle, I had to push thoughts of him ever returning to surgery far out of my mind. But I soothed my mind with the notion that the College of Surgeons would have experienced cases like this before, and we will have a pathway back already laid out. We had already come a long way, and on November 13, I resolved to not care whether Siva ever returned to surgery. At that moment, seeing Siva walk over to greet his visitors was heartwarming enough. We resolved to focus on the present and let the future unfold as it would.

Discharge

Prema

We had waited for discharge day for what felt like so long—a day when we could exit through the hospital doors and back into our world. Knowing how much care Siva had needed in the hospital, I resolved to hire a personal support worker. Our housekeeper's husband David was available and was perfect to fill this role. I quickly began organizing accessories to use at home—a cane, a wheelchair—any assistive devices that would help Siva get through his day.

Discharge on December 1, 2017, marked nine long weeks of appointments, hope, hopelessness, and waiting. For me, it also entailed maintaining a semblance of my usual routines. I had been juggling work with Siva's ever-evolving needs. At home, we had dutiful children supporting us with our ever-faithful dog. There were light bulbs that needed to be changed, chores that needed to be completed, and leaves that needed to be raked. These mundane activities and support from our children comforted us, especially Siva—his only request had been for our children to continue to focus on their studies to "make Appa happy."

However, "making Appa happy" after discharge was not always easy. The safety net provided by twenty-four seven caregivers was removed, and we transitioned into leading a new charge on life at home on our own.

You name it, we threw it at Siva, and some days he threw it back in tiredness and frustration. Outpatient rehab, driving rehab, golfing rehab, personal trainer workouts, acupuncture, chiropractor appointments—we even throw in a Yanni concert. How quickly we forgot that we were all in mourning for a former life and were merely filling our days with activities that kept our minds from straying to realities and places that we did not want to go to.

Christmas 2017 came and went in a wave of busyness and disbelief. We are Hindus so for Christmas in our home we made our own traditions without the religious celebration. We made it about being together as a family and exchanging gifts. On Christmas morning before gifts are exchanged, Siva as the head of the family would say a few words. This message he designs based on what has happened the past year and where we are as a family and what to aspire for the coming year. As this message is imparted once a year, it can be quite impactful especially to the children. This year was different. Siva talked about his predicament and thanked us for remaining strong and emphasized to his children that they should stay on course with their life and aspirations. The gifts we exchanged were thoughtful. My children got their dad a virtual simulator, a PlayStation VR, which they thought would help his hand-eye coordination and spatial orientation as part of his rehabilitation. I tried my best to create the same atmosphere at home as we have had every year during Christmas. We were happy to be home but couldn't quite believe how we got to this familiar but new frontier. We looked ahead in the hope that 2018 would be better.

After all that we had been through in the past few months, we decided to bring some normalcy to our lives and planned a trip to warmer climates. It seemed like it might be just what the doctor ordered. So, Siva and I ordered a trip to the Bahamas, followed shortly after by a family trip to Portugal, easing ourselves into a new year and a new era. Siva flew with assistance and was transported through the airport hallways in style. Flying was easy, and the breaks away were nice, but they were covering up the cracks, and we were not even coming close to looking at the underlying current that we knew was coming. In dark moments, Siva shared that he couldn't comprehend why it had all happened to him. Remembering that his mother nearly died giving birth to him, he wondered often if he was cursed or if he was born evil and that the stroke was payback for misdemeanours in another life. At other times he talked about evil forces that may have hexed him. He just was still grappling with the fact that how could this have happened.

As the year passed, midway through 2018, Siva began to think about the idea of retraining. First, there was a constant grappling with what other career options he might have if he couldn't be a surgeon again. Many ideas passed through his mind quickly, and at one point, we really thought that he might get into investing or day-trading. I knew that none of the options would make him happy and wasn't what he truly wanted. So, we began to think about retraining Siva's brain and movements so that he could return to being a surgeon. A senior colleague and friend at the university told Siva about different options available to him and that he couldn't see any reasons as to why he couldn't return to surgery someday, after a lot of effort, work, retraining, and practice. Siva immediately began to try the simulators for endoscopy and laparoscopy in CSTAR, a surgical skills lab in London. Each session was $200, and the 1.25-hour drive back and forth became tiring. Striving to be the ever-dutiful, supportive wife and fellow surgeon, I created a surgical simulation model at home.

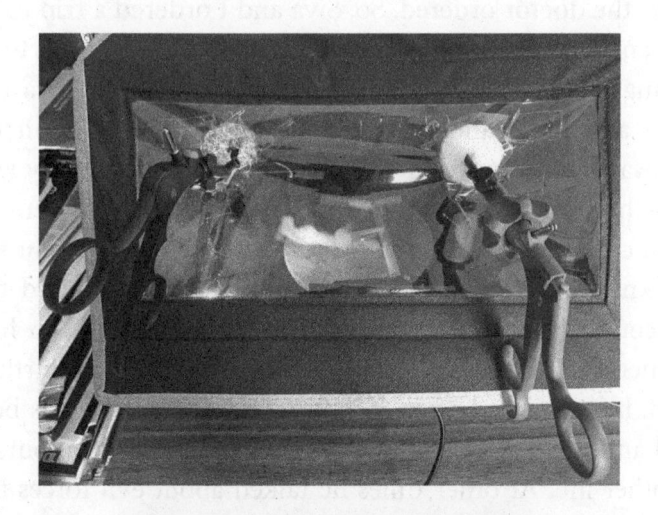

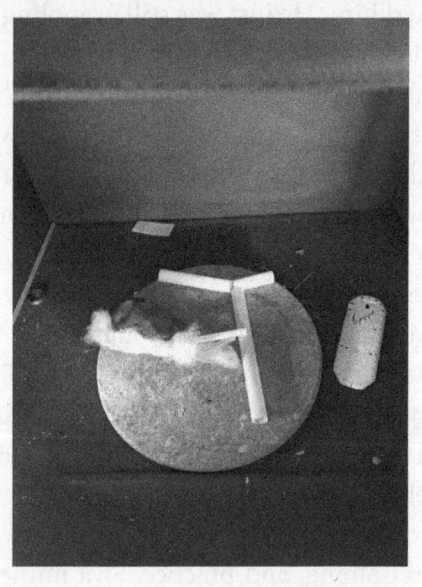

The Journey of Two Surgeons Through Stroke

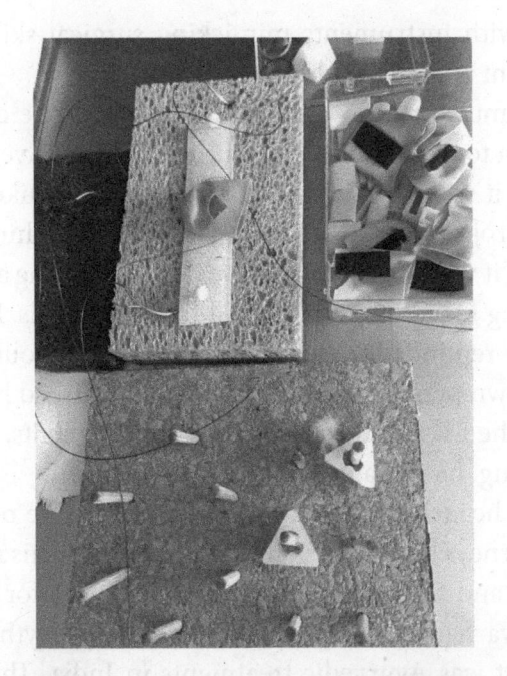

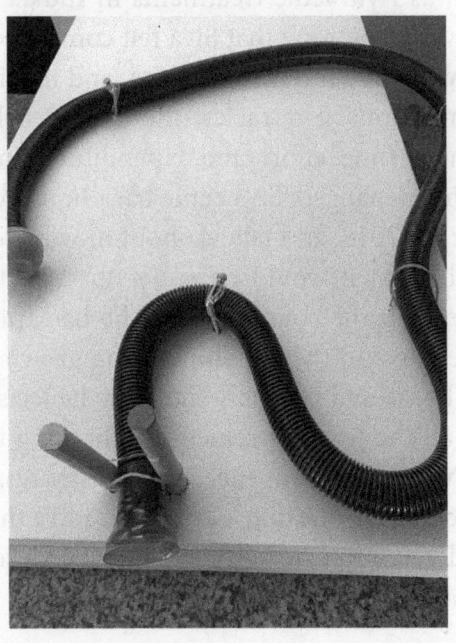

This with instruments mimicking surgical skills was to enable him to retrain at home.

The simulator was rudimentary but could be effective if used. Siva took a look, touched it, and then resolved to practice with it someday, maybe. It sat in his study like a school science project. I often wondered if I had made him feel like a child. If it were me, I would have been practicing and trying everything I could to re-hone and refine my skills. But I continuously reminded myself that this was not about me. Siva was his own person, and despite how diminished he seemed lying in the ER and through all the appointments, prodding and pulling, he was a proud man and surgeon.

As we headed into months eleven and twelve poststroke, Siva's journeys began. First, he headed home to his mother in Malaysia and from there to India. In his quest for improvement, Siva had decided that he would try anything. First on his list was Ayurvedic treatments in India. This type of treatment was something that Siva felt connected to, a treatment involving herbal remedies, yoga, and meditations. The practitioner promised miracles, the patient believed them and after much time, effort, and expenditure, nothing much seemed to have changed. Siva came back home to our family on October 13, 2018, and talked about moving to India long term. He thought it would be easier for him to return to practice there, in the country where he had trained, where he knew people and the system. Having grown up there, it is truly his home and probably the place he feels most comfortable in all the world. I remember thinking to myself, If he goes, it will be without me, as I had my responsibilities here—two children, one dog, one house, and a thriving practice. I wondered if our new frontier included a separation as husband and wife.

Way Back When

Siva—Recounted April 27, 2019

Growing up in Malaysia, I observed my hard-working parents going about their busy lives, my mother as a teacher, and my father as a court interpreter. They had an arranged marriage, but not until after my mother had attended university and teacher training, gaining a Bachelor of Arts and a position teaching at a secondary school. My parents moved around Malaysia frequently, enjoying new experiences and challenges, eventually culminating with my mother teaching at a university and my father working at a courthouse.

My mother is one of six children. Her father, my maternal grandfather, was a moneylender and revered businessman. My grandmother focused on raising her family, but her brain was made for numbers and computing—she was sharp and quick with numbers, weights, and fractions. Her brain was perfectly tuned for the market trading and bartering system in which she grew up. I'm not sure why my grandfather sent my mother to university; he must have seen something in her. This was in Malaysia in the 1950s, where a woman attending university and working were unusual and ground-breaking achievements. I think that is where my forging spirit came from—it was inherited, not created.

My Burmese-born father spoke seven languages: Tamil, Japanese, Malay, English, and three Indian dialects. Here I am, a man of few words. I prefer to observe, ponder, and act; verbalizing, I leave to others. That is how it has always been.

I was born on November 20, 1960. Bringing me into the world, my mother had a difficult birth and very nearly died. Due to my safe arrival and my mother's survival, my grandfather saw me as blessed and a force for good luck. I was born his favourite, and that is how I was raised and treated. I was the oldest and naughtiest of three boys, and together with my brothers Bala and Jeya, we gave our parents a run for their money.

One of my earliest memories of life with my parents was heading out on the weekend in our black Morris Minor car. I sat in the back full of anticipation of the many fruits we would savour at the weekend market. A dollar would buy 100 rambutans—a hairy-skinned fruit that filled our car and our stomachs. Rambutans are hailed as super fruits—rich in calcium, potassium, and magnesium and full of vitamins B2, B3, and C. Their antioxidant and anticancer properties are now widely recognized. However, to four-year-old Siva, they were just deliciousness on my lips and in my mouth. Super fruits for super Siva. Perhaps the stores of goodness were built up in me, and when my reserves were depleted or my luck ran out, the stroke wheedled its way into my right brain.

When I was nine, my grandfather asked me if I would like to move to India and live with him; naturally, I said yes. I was his favourite; he was mine. Together, we went to inform my parents of my move, 2,600 kilometres away across the ocean. Not once did I question the move, nor did I fear it. Not me, not Siva. Siva was born to break new ground. Leaving my brothers behind didn't even enter my mind, for I, special Siva, was embarking on an adventure with a beloved grandfather.

I'm sure that my mother must've been saddened by my decision to move from Malaysia to India, for I would only return to her during the summer holidays. I never really went back to live with her again. She knew that this was an opportunity not to be turned down and that questioning her father was not a prudent thing to do.

I was excited to head into a new adventure and be close to my cousins. I was quite happy because I was my grandfather's favourite grandson. Once I arrived in India, I did miss my parents, but school and local activities helped me quickly forget my parents and my brothers. I lived in the moment as I continue to do to this day.

I arrived in the little village of Kandadevi, South India, to live among cousins running barefoot and cow herders living simple but contented lives. The St. Mary's Catholic school to which I was sent for year five was five kilometres away. My memory is that I ran to school every day, dressed in a white shirt and khaki shorts, with the purpose of travelling rather than merely arriving. There were so many stops and detours to experience along the way: paddy fields, a Catholic church with praying styles akin to practicing exorcisms, a brick factory—so much wonder and industry for a young boy to observe and explore during his first year in a new country. I was surrounded by aunts and uncles and brother-and-sister-cousins. My life was full of action and busyness.

Year six in school brought change, and a boarding school north of Chennai was my new frontier. My mother knew the nuns at the boarding school, and they were only too happy to take me on for their acquaintances. My uniform was maroon and white in colour, and it felt akin to a suit of armour. Here

I was, far away from family, the village and freedom, relying on infrequent visits from my beloved grandfather to lighten the day. My grandfather came to visit me, proud that his chosen one was excelling at school. I learned to adapt, to adopt a stiff upper lip, to never complain, but to get on with the project and task at hand. Under pressure conditions, diamonds are fashioned.

The boys at boarding school became like family, and we shared a need for fun, love, and security... oh, and mischief, too. We frequently irritated the school's gardener. I vividly remember one day making a mess in an area he had worked hard to tidy up. He chased after us, but I managed to evade him, swinging from bar to bar on a climbing frame until my luck ran out. Down I crashed onto my wrists, breaking my right one. The pain seared through me, but I'm sure it was nothing compared to the horror that flowed through the gardener; I could see the fear of potential job loss in his eyes. The school took me to a traditional bone setter, who massaged oils into my arm and cajoled it back into place before splinting it. My right wrist was set to heal perfectly, but not before I howled with pain. Perhaps my right side has always been weaker. First, a weak wrist, and then a fragile right brain.

As I sat years later, with scientific and fact-based knowledge in hand, I celebrated how a traditional bonesetter, without the benefits of X-rays, could feel his way to put me and my bones back together. Closing your eyes and feeling what's right, rather than looking for what's right, symbolized how I felt about how my life was heading after my stroke. Feeling the way forward versus seeing it—how spiritual that is. How in keeping with Siva's being.

Scaling Great Heights to a Stroke

Siva

Base camp is perhaps where my stroke started. My desire to breach frontiers may have opened up some weaknesses in my right brain.

In May 2017, four months before my stroke, I conquered Mount Kailash in Tibet, 21,778 feet above sea level. I didn't conquer it in the sense of planting a flag on the summit—for that has never been achieved—but I did pilgrimage there, like people have done for thousands of years. Kailash is sacred for pilgrims, and Hindus believe that circling Mount Kailash on foot in a clockwise direction is a holy ritual that will bring good fortune.

Did it bring me good fortune? Pushing my body beyond its frontiers at high altitudes may have exposed fissures and allowed weakness to creep in. The climb itself was equal parts grueling and exhilarating and was everything that

I had dreamed of, and perhaps lived for: Siva the pioneer, always pushing to new frontiers.

In preparation for the climb, I had worked hard for months, less on my fitness and more on my breathing. I rose at 4:30 a.m. every day to work on gaining control over my breathing. Using the yoga techniques that I had learned in India thirty-five years prior, I learned to survive on less oxygen. As we climbed Mount Kailash, the fittest climbers failed while I succeeded.

In hindsight, the discipline it took to achieve this feat was staggering. Post-stroke, the discipline needed to do exercises that enhanced my gait, my mind and my endurance eluded me. I was unsure as to what I was training for. What was my purpose?

Prema created lists for me: endless lists. But there they sat on paper. They were not my lists. I just wanted to get back to normal, or rather my new normal, and I believed that doing surgeries would rectify everything and give me everything I needed. Prema created a mock surgical framework for me to practice on. It was very clever, but it looked ridiculous and made me feel like a child. Yes, I knew that I should have been preparing and should have been better prepared. Not preparing made me feel guilty but watching Netflix for hours on end each day became my guilty pleasure. Prema despaired, and I flicked deftly through the channels with my trusty right hand.

So, what was stopping me? I say that it wasn't fear of failure. I rationalized my inertia by suggesting that the outcome would be what it would be, regardless of how well I prepared. When I heard myself say this out loud, I knew that it didn't make sense, but I couldn't explain my thinking. My brain was damaged. It was the stroke. I needed to get back.

I thought that perhaps getting back might look like new adventures. Once, I had entertained thoughts of becoming more spiritually aware and ran away from medical school in India to study and practice yoga, eschewing meat to become more at one with the world. The yogis told me that my future was bright, but my parents and grandfather were aghast when they learned of my new adventure. They brought me home, fed me meat, and reset my direction.

As I sat and pondered what the future held, my thoughts wandered to yoga, asanas, and spirituality. I remember wondering deeply: Is that what I need to get back to? That path was somewhat forbidden to me, but at the time, I now had a choice. Certainly, I wanted my licence to practice medicine back, but I really wanted a licence to be me: a Siva without restrictions, limitations, boundaries, or supervision—out and away from under watchful eyes. The Siva that was meant to be. I made it to Mount Kailash, but what I was going through post-stroke—that was my Everest.

Thinking about the enormity of everything made the muscles in my left arm freeze. It took a lot of concentration and brain power to overcome the lock to free the movement. So instead of concentrating on complicated thoughts about my life and future, I had to concentrate on something so fundamental. It was tiring. But there it was. Once, I had been disciplined enough to gain control over my breathing.

I had a moment where I wondered, what if spiritual discipline, breathing, mindfulness, and meditation could help me make basic movements routine and mundane again? I planned to practice that. Later. After Netflix.

Get Back to Where You Once Belonged

Siva—Recounted March 16, 2019

Returning to work was hard. I voluntarily declared the stroke to the College of Surgeons and Physicians of Ontario, assuming that they had established pathways laid out to assist a surgeon with a return to work. I was wrong. The College of Physicians and Surgeons of Ontario (CPSO) had no return-to-work protocols, so I was setting a template and was a pioneer once again.

I consulted with a CPSO-appointed neurologist who did a full assessment and declared that I was good cognitively, but that an assessment to report on my surgical abilities could only be made by another surgeon. Thus, I had to prove that I could perform my surgical skills safely and would require a supervisor to assess me. I was confident that my colleagues, with whom I had worked and collaborated for ten years, would help with this assessment.

Returning to work was the sole focus of my life, but it was just one of many things for my colleagues at the hospital. There were countless licensing issues and delays, and patiently and skillfully navigating them was a pioneering journey. My mission was to be declared a most responsible physician (MRP) for my patients again—someone I have always been as a person and a physician. But there was no easily navigable path back, and it was sobering to think that in physician circles, I might never be an MRP again. I accepted that I might always be supervised.

How did I feel? Angry. Angry with the situation, with the stroke and with the delays in paperwork to start the process for me to return to work. For me, those roadblocks and delays were just checks and balances for a hospital board of administration and for surgeons in a litigious world.

Everyone was fearful of the consequences. Patient care and safety are paramount, as they have always been and continue to be for me. I felt confident that I would know my limitations. I just needed to try, to feel what it was like to stand poised for surgery.

If this was the end of MRP status for me, that was probably okay. I didn't really mind being supervised; however, I did mind not being given the chance to prove that I could come back.

Cognitively, I was clear—my tests confirmed this. But why was there this lingering doubt for everyone? We live in a world where the physical overrides the mental—where physical limitations trump a fully functioning mind. Stephen Hawking lived this.

Independent assessments would be made by another surgeon so that there was no bias of judgement about my abilities—as if any self-respecting medic would run the risk of damaging their reputation. If this was the Malaysia of my youth and training, we would just get someone into the operating room (OR) to supervise them and see how they do. Not in Canada, though—I understood this, but it still frustrated me. Prema said it would be the same in Malaysia now; no one would risk their reputation.

In Malaysia, I operated as a general surgeon, carrying out both mundane and complex surgeries. Every day was different and exciting, with adrenaline pumping. In Canada, life has been more predictable. General surgeons, despite their title, actually specialize here. I focused on endoscopies, doing twenty-five a day! Having no licence to practice and a CPSO record that stated I have "ceased to practice medicine"—what was my life status now? Where was my purpose? What was my purpose?

If I could get my licence restored, I thought, I could get back in the OR, and a world of options would open up to me. Maybe I would volunteer overseas; maybe I would become a locum in the great white north of Canada. So many "maybes," but to me, maybes were options, choices, and decisions that had to be made—all things that had been taken out of my hands eighteen months before by my stroke.

After two years "out of practice," the CPSO dictated that I would have to return to do exams, to recertify—back to the beginning, again. I would have been a junior surgeon three times, first when training in Malaysia, second when we moved to Canada, and third when I returned post-stroke. Three times lucky or just plain unfair?

I just needed to get back. I still had my parking bay at the hospital. It seemed a small price to pay for a connection to my former life. Every Tuesday, I attended surgical team meetings at the hospital—I attended every week after my stroke. It was a way for me to keep my hand in the game as well as a way for my colleagues to assess me, and I know that beneath the smiles and behind the handshakes, they were curious. How was I moving? How was my mind? How had Siva changed? And here was the irony. While my left hand may not have functioned with quite the same finesse as it once did, my brain's computing power felt uncompromised eighteen months post-stroke. These colleagues still sought my input and professional opinion on complex cases. They knew how I functioned as a high-performing general surgeon, sometimes finding ways to fix the unfixable. However, as time went by, my opinions became less important, and I did not feel that my presence was valued. I stopped attending these meetings in 2019.

I just needed to get back, I remember thinking to myself. But how would I feel when I got the call to say, "Siva, you're back on the roster," Fear? No. Nervous? Yes. I was to be heading into a three- to four-month assessment and would be under a microscope. Everything I did, every move I made or didn't make, would be watched, monitored, scrutinized, recorded, and documented. Siva was to be a specimen under the bright OR lights. Little slip-ups that every surgeon makes along the way and then deftly corrects would be labelled deficits and shortcomings. They would be things that I did wrong because of the stroke. I'd never had anyone to blame before; it had always been down to me. Now I had this "thing" that underwrote everything I did and spoke. If I was sad, it was the stroke. If I was angry, it was the stroke. In surgery, if I made a minor mistake, it would be because of the stroke. A stroke that had changed Siva, that had taken away his ability. Siva would not be the surgeon he once was. Yes, I would be an MRP once again but not at the pinnacle of the OR mountain. Instead, I would be back at base camp. Base camp was still quite high, though.

Prema

The day Siva's notification from the CPSO arrived is clear in my mind.

To see "ceased to practice medicine" was shocking in black and white. The college had not received some paperwork and so had made this determination. It felt like a death notification. The end. A cancer diagnosis would have been easier to deal with and fight. There would have been a clear course of treatment to follow, with reasonably predictable outcomes. Stroke is different. It's wilier, and the same stroke in two people can have polar opposite impacts. I hid the CPSO letter. Siva would be upset, I thought, and I wanted to protect him from what was another blow, another injustice on the road back to work. Here I was, mother and wife to Siva.

I kept the CPSO letter tucked away, but I could feel it in the house. There was incessant noise from the television. Netflix and F1 racing blared, but nothing was louder than Siva's silence. With the week's list untouched, a drive in the country provided welcome relief and a purpose to our Saturday. The children were coming home for a visit, and we were to have a nice family meal. The house would be busy, and for a while, we would forget about the stroke and work and just enjoy each other's company. I reminded myself that Siva would make progress and that all would be well in the world. Not making progress was my biggest fear for me and for Siva.

With Siva, everything has always been about making progress. Our lives in Malaysia were established, our children were thriving, and family was around, but Siva wanted to breach new frontiers. That's how we came to Canada. A bridging program for physicians opened up temporarily and offered a window of opportunity, presenting a passage to a new frontier, country, and continent. Siva seized the opportunity, and I was pleased to follow along. The opportunities for our two children were better in Canada. It must have been fate that this fissure opened up to us, as it allowed Siva to be a general surgeon and for me to be an ENT surgeon specialist.

I was actually prepared to do whatever it took to get our family settled, even if that meant not working. However, Siva insisted that my career path continue uninterrupted, which is quite enlightening to reflect on for someone who grew up in a world where women played second fiddle to men, always.

The bridging program opportunity closed suddenly behind us, which truly made it another fissure in our lives. A moment to seize an opportunity.

Prema as Sherpa

Prema

Lists, plans, goals, appointments, more lists and searching. But what were we searching for? What was I searching for? Everything had changed; there was no denying that. The future was once full of promise, and then it seemed so daunting. I had often thought that Siva would go through this return-to-work journey and then return in whatever capacity he could, and only then would life turn out close to what it had been. I think I built that roadmap based on all that we knew and the home and office that we loved.

Things did not seem so daunting first thing in the morning as the warm water of the shower washed over me. There was hope and possibility as it washed away fears and calmed worries. To this day, when I can grab those lightbulb moments and release myself from the stress of a life-altering event, anything seems possible.

I remember thinking, what if I broke away from all the preconceived ideas and said, "Hey, let's see what happens or does not. What if we are prepared to uproot ourselves, relocate, or maybe downsize and start a new life where we both can reboot? This roadmap is exciting and gives life a whole new perspective." My stress levels dropped, and I felt excited looking toward the future.

I thought it wouldn't matter if Siva never returned to the hospital; it wouldn't matter that we would have to set off for fresh woods and pastures. Siva climbed mountains before, and this time, I told myself, I would be his Sherpa, rising before dawn to prepare us for the hike.

I felt different in those moments. The more I let go, the more in control I felt. It was bizarre that I was giving up on going back, but it was liberating. Because I accepted the fact that things would never be the same as they once were, and that was okay. Siva has always been a workaholic. When he was working, he was exhausted at the end of each day; there was no time to just sit and be.

Post-stroke, and to this day, we sit, we eat together, we go for drives in the country, and we go to the grocery store together. We are together now, but our days for quite a while were very different. My routine was largely unchanged, but everything was different. The office was different: no Siva. The hospital was different: no Siva. The parking lot was different: no Siva. So here I was, the same but going without. A stroke that had divided Siva's brain had brought us together, but Siva had moved on, and it was I who had been left behind.

We started some return-to-work steps for Siva and began the process with CPSO, the Canadian Medical Protective Association (CMPA), and the hospital. We soon learned that there were no established precedents for post-stroke surgeons. There was no back-to-work road map that had already been laid out by the governing bodies.

We were alone on this road with our lawyer from CMPA representing us with communications to CPSO and the hospital management. Siva reached out to the Royal College of Surgeons to see if they had any resources for him, but it was a circular journey, and they referred him back to CPSO. Siva had to be a trail blazer and set out his own plan. He had to work with so many layers of several regulatory bodies and relied heavily on his fellow surgeon colleagues at work.

Siva returned to Malaysia in early December 2018 to tend to his sick mother. How ironic that he returned to his mother as a caregiver when he himself needed care and nurturing. However, how joyful it was to be able to spend time with her as she went through cancer treatments. If he had not had a stroke, he would have been far too busy to spend this time with his mother. While there, he investigated obtaining a licence to practice and realized that time had moved on and that it was not going to be the easy feat he had imagined.

I tended to the house and work in the three long months that Siva was away. He had moved on and out; his family had been left behind. We made the most of it and enjoyed our Christmas as best we could. The bell tolled in my ear for the end of a marriage; I had no choice but to block it out—that would have been way too much to take.

Siva returned to us on March 2, 2019. Jet lag was combined with grumpiness and malaise, followed by news that the many delays in processing Siva's paperwork had resulted in the College of Surgeons' website stating that Dr. Murugappan had ceased to practice medicine. Devastating.

The daily wait to hear something positive—a sliver of something that would give us some hope that Siva might return to work—was tedious. We knew that what we were trying to do meant that we would have to forge a path for Siva, and that would mean heartache, frustration, and hurdles along the way. Some days, negativity invaded me, and I lost hope that there would be a brave new world. What was the point of all this struggle? I was living in a half-world with a husband who seemed half-committed to our marriage. Other days, I could quash the groundswell and know that, as long as we were together, we would be prepared for every eventuality along our journey.

Towards the end of March 2019, we learned that Siva's return date to work under supervision at the hospital was set for June 3, 2019. It seemed like a long, long way off, and I wondered if Siva had the patience to wait or whether we should try to expedite it. Surprisingly, he was okay with it. Having a start date in a process that had been riddled with bumps and disappointments gave him something to work towards. I looked at him and wondered how he would survive in that harsh climate. Did *I* want him to return more than *he* did? People were still asking me how Siva was doing; they hadn't seen much of him and were curious. Was he disabled? Would he return to work?

The bottom line was that Siva was confident that he could perform the most routine and elective procedures. Phew, that was a relief. At least he had that much confidence and optimism, because if I had to provide him that boost, too, it would have been too hard. I was beginning to feel like I was running dry from worrying about him, about my son and what lay ahead for him in his career, and my mother-in-law, who was still struggling with the effects of radiation on her throat.

A beautiful spring morning and a walk with our dog, Benji, replenished my spirits. I sat in the backyard, bundled up from the cold, with the sun shining on my face with Benji, my little angel, by my feet. He had been by my side for over that past year and a half. I think God places little angels with us. Benji, to this day, is still mine.

Patience, Patients, Patience, Patients

Siva

My mantra during those long days at home was just one word: *patience*. On brighter days, when I would look ahead to getting back to work, it was *patients*—the focus of my life. I missed my routines and my patients. What was my purpose, if not to be a surgeon? Was being a husband, father, son, and friend enough? Are these the things that define life's purpose?

On days when the OR was beyond my grasp, my mantra was *patience*. If I sat still long enough, if I reignited the spirituality that Prema was trying hard to encourage, would life's purpose reveal itself to me?

For so long after the stroke, there were only three things that I wanted to do.

1. Get my licence back: that gave me options and choices.

2. Get back to me: that allowed me to measure and assess what I was capable of.

3. Run: this was a new frontier and not something I had ever done.

Now, there was a fourth thing to add to the list.

4. Find my purpose: this would allow me to be Siva.

Since my stroke, my brain had rewired and forced me to focus on doing simple things. The synapses had been working hard to try to get me to the point where doing simple things was second nature. How terrifying it was to have to admit that and say it out loud. If it was true, then I had reached the path to enlightenment. An appreciation for the complexity and beauty of the simple is to be in a state of Zen.

Patience, patience, patience.

Children

Prema

I worried about Siva all the time. Seeing his slow movements in the grocery store made me fearful about how he would function back in the OR. This couldn't be a one-act play for him. This was real, and he would be closely watched, under a microscope—and no one looked good under one of those. I asked myself, What if he failed? How would that set him back? Getting back, getting back to our routines, getting back to our lives—that was what we both wanted. I wrote lists for Siva, filled with suggestions for how he might spend his time while I was at work and in surgery. Lumosity challenges, setting time aside for surgical simulations, time for exercise, time for movement. It was like having two jobs; rather, it was more like having three or four. The lists went unchecked and maybe even unread. Really, they were my lists, my steps for getting Siva back. I forgot that Siva always forges his own path.

Siva could not see how much had changed from my perspective and how different I felt about work and life. My life had changed dramatically since his stroke. But in a way that was probably so keenly yet quietly observed by Siva, it had not changed at all—for I still walked out the door every day to operate and consult. I wondered if Siva was envious of that. Every morning, I would leave the house and drive the bends in the road that snake the shape of the river. Within ten minutes, I was as far away from the stroke as it was possible to be as I walked through the hospital or consulting room doors. Then, my life resumed.

When the bright lights in the OR room are switched on, we are truly on stage in a theatre. I become the leading actor, and even if I mess up on where to stand or forget a few lines, my skills and confidence allow me to rectify and readjust. The audience and other performers barely notice. It wasn't going to be like that for Siva. He would be in the spotlight and scrutinized.

Our children were away at university, but since the stroke, I had found a new child. Siva, whether during the nine weeks in hospital or from the time he came home, needed care, food, company, and encouragement. I set little tasks for him and offered comfort and encouragement, but none of it seemed to reach the part of him that was lost. It made me sad to look at Siva, to witness his journey, and to see how it had taken away his purpose. I wished I had had the stroke, for maybe we would have coped better.

Encouraging Siva was something I did a lot of—encouraged him to seek alternative therapies, to try new things such as Tai Chi, to visit India, to spend time with his mother in Malaysia, to write, to find a purpose. Anything to help him. He is five years my senior. I respect him in every way, and I have followed him halfway around the world to Canada. We are opposites: he is quiet; I like to talk. He likes to do very little; I like to be on the move. Life for us is like a seesaw, but we operate in absolute harmony. We are joined together, moving as counterweights in opposite directions. In unison, there is balance, so since the stroke, we had been trying to find what weight we could both bear, what weights to add or let go of.

Fit to Go Back

Siva—Recounted April 14, 2019

Not that I was counting, but there we were, sixty days in. Finally, there were some positive developments that set me on course and back to surgery. So, with the news that my colleagues were willing to supervise me and having signed the necessary paperwork and undertakings for the CPSO, the preparation work to build my endurance and stamina, my fitness and sharpness had started in earnest. I knew it was something I should have been working on long ago, but I just couldn't start. There was no purpose back then, and every time I began to think about the journey back, we experienced another setback.

I am not sure what kick-started me that week. But, like the day of the stroke, something inside me shifted. Three trips to the YMCA for independent workouts on the bicycle and walking tracks. Sessions with my personal trainer. Rehab sessions for stroke patients. The improvement in my mood and appearance was immediate, and people commented on it. I slept better than I had done in a long time as I recalibrated and reset my body clock.

They say that positivity breeds positivity. I think that, during that week, this was true. Because I closed out the week with a text message that changed everything...

The CPSO said I was fit to return under supervision. Through a text message to Prema, we learned that the medical advisory council at the hospital agreed and said I was fit to return. The surgical supervisors who were to be reporting back to CPSO on my progress held my life in their hands. I wondered if they realized that. For so long, we had been peers and colleagues, some of whom I had aided with complex cases. Now I was relying on them to help me get my licence back. So, a simple text message from my colleague was loaded with significance for me, for Prema, and for our future.

How did I feel when I received the news that they were preparing for my return? The response was as complex as the stroke itself: excitement, relief, hope, but evident too was fear that I masked as apathy. Did I really want to go back after such a long time? Did I want to go back to the grind? Did I want to be put to the test again? Maybe I felt guilty, too. Here I was pushing to go back and pulling to stay away.

There was another life available to Siva, one in which he used the word "no" more often. If life is a pie and time is the slices allocated to different parts of our lives, then I had some decisions to make about how I sliced the pie. The pre-stroke pie had only three slices: work, sleep, and golf. I was so proud of my ability to work long hours, to get by on little sleep or food, or water or self-care. Powering through twenty to twenty-five scopes a day was exhilarating then, being on call and responding promptly, never saying "no"—those were all things I valued. Hardly surprising, then, that I drove myself to the precipice. I always thought that my heart would give out before my vascular system. The stroke shocked me, and while something shifted internally that day, something undefinable shifted, too—was it my wakeup call?

My work life was geared to service, service to my patients, to my colleagues, and to my community. Prema described me as a workaholic, and I was proud of that. Being a surgeon is about being the best, doing the best—that is how I was trained, to show no weakness, no tiredness, and to always power through. Never once did I feel burdened by this role and these responsibilities; instead, I thrived on them. I see now that I set the tone for how my world operated. Fast-paced decision-making, reliance on immediate updates from nurses, secretaries, responsive to patient needs—all squeezing and fitting in more and more patients, more and more work. Service, service, service above everything else. Better than the rest. Frontiers. Vanguards.

However, the rules of the game had changed. Actually, I think the game itself had changed. Siva would not make such fast-paced decisions; he wouldn't need to initiate, as he would be assisting other surgeons. They would lead, and Siva would follow. Assuming that all would go well, that I was assessed by my colleagues and a third-party evaluator and deemed to be competent and capable, I would undoubtedly return to my former pace. Right back in. At least that's how I thought of it. My mind was guiding me to places I sometimes didn't want to go. One minute I saw the other slices of the pie, the next I saw just one big pie, with no slices and "work" tattooed into the crust.

After months of observing, thinking, pondering, reflecting, and spending time on my own, the pie slices were looking greatly different. The new pie would be sliced to carve out dedicated time for my family and for doing things other than work, and there would be a slice for time to think. Now that I was on this train, I thought I should probably make a slice for Netflix, too!

A former surgeon and colleague were amazed by my desire to get back into the fray. He had stepped away from full-time work and had carved up his life into many different pieces. Surgery remained a component, but it was not the sole one. Mixed in were activities like day-trading, golf, travel, and time with family. I guess the difference between us is that he chose to step away from the OR and it was forced upon me. I didn't see it coming, even though I drove myself there. I never predicted or planned for a day when surgery would not be a part of my life. So, the stroke and all that it took away was a shock, and I still can't believe that it happened to me. Retirement was not, is not, on my radar; I still have frontiers to breach. At the top of my game, being cut down and redirected was such a cruel blow to me: me, who had worked harder than most other people, me who had thrived in that high-performance environment.

With the approval of the hospital's medical advisory council to return to the OR, the next step was the hospital's board approval, which would rubberstamp my return. It should have been routine approval if my surgeon peers were ready to receive me. With all the legal checks and balances in place, all that was left to do was sign the bottom line to make it happen. On darker days, it felt like the world was conspiring against me. On brighter days, I appreciated my colleagues' efforts to get me back. Their time was valuable, their reputations were on the line, and their patient care levels and scores were of the utmost importance. They knew me, who I was and what I was capable of. But let's face it. No one knew what the new me was capable of under the bright lights, least of all me.

Prema

So many questions filled my mind. Could we bring the hospital board meeting forward? Who might be prepared to do us a favour and ask the question for us? Did we want to call in favours? Was Siva even ready if they did?

That week, I was glad that Siva's energy had returned. He was revitalized, and I hoped he could carry some of the disappointment that I had willingly carried for so long. Work, patients, children, school, home, yard work, pets, changing light bulbs, worrying for everyone, making "to-do" lists for everyone. This week, I was tired. Tired of being a type A.

Waiting Game

Siva—Recounted June 2, 2019

The days of May 2019 were long. I understood that my surgeon colleagues who agreed to supervise my work had to ensure that they knew just what they were agreeing to. The days ticked by slowly until the formality of a hospital board meeting was set to approve my return. I sat at home and thought. Too much time to think is never good, so it led me to worry. What if someone on the board, a nonmedical person, questioned my return? Who would advocate for me? I, who had no status and who was reliant on benevolence, on the faith that my years of being a good colleague and surgeon would stand to me and count for something.

The Ontario College of Surgeons had approved my return, the medical advisory committee at the hospital had approved my return, and the credentialing committee of the hospital board had approved my return. Now the hospital's board of directors needed to place their seal of approval.

But such was my worry that we would hit another obstacle, I urged Prema to set a meeting with a friend familiar with the process. We met at a local Tim Hortons, which seemed like such an incongruous place to discuss all that had dominated my thoughts since the day of the stroke. The coffee was as warm as the meeting, and we candidly discussed the upcoming board meeting and my fears. It was during this chat that it really dawned on me just how much the team at the hospital had done to get me back. They had checked in on me, included me in weekly meetings, sought my advice, took the unprecedented and unknown step of agreeing to supervise me, and they were standing for me at the board meeting, vouching for me. The weight of holding all my worries had been heavy, weighing me down and clouding my judgment on occasion.

The board meeting was set for 5:00 p.m. on May 30, 2019. This was eighteen months since my stroke. I was at home waiting with Benji, our family dog and my constant companion. Prema was at work. She was waiting for 5:00 p.m., but as it turned out, a child with a split lip needed her surgical attention, and she was in the OR. Had I acted like a child with a pouty lip sometimes? Most likely, but Prema had never pointed it out. Instead, she had been my voice when I was mute and my voice of reason when I could only scream. Just after 5:30 p.m., Prema called to share the news. The board had approved my return. This was the news we had waited for so long. Prema hung up. I opened a bottle of wine and stared at Benji. After so long a fight, it was almost anticlimactic. But I drank the glass of wine, for this was a day to celebrate all that had been and all that would be. Now it was time for me to get back to the grind.

Prema

We all had doubts. Who wouldn't have, given all the ups, downs, and hurdles we had faced and jumped through. As the end of the May board meeting approached, I reached out to my colleagues at the hospital for advice. I questioned whether we should try to expedite the board meeting date. "No" was the resounding answer. To us, every day was a long day of waiting, and to them, it flew by with appointments and consultations. So, another few weeks of waiting were clocked up to the journey. Everyone still told me how much they missed Siva. I was the conduit to him, whether by text, email, or verbal messages. That was how it had been since the stroke. Since Siva had come home from rehab, he had largely been out of sight. My role was to make sure that he was never out of mind. I diligently answered all the questions and responded to all the messages; I was a voice for Siva when he fell silent.

The closer the date for the board meeting came, the closer questions and doubts bubbled to the surface. All the "what ifs." Who will be Siva's advocate? I messaged a friend in the hopes of learning more about the process. In a Tim Hortons coffee shop, I got my answers.

May 30, 2019, rolled around and along with it the worry, terror, and heartbreak for Siva's fate. A bust lip on a child kept me in surgery and away from my phone for the first part of the board meeting. I stopped the bleeding—both of the lip and in my heart. There was work to be done and lives to be saved, and that was where I turned my focus.

At 5:30 p.m., my text message alert beeped. There they were: a few short words that we had waited so long to see. Siva's return was approved by the board. The nurses in the OR, all of whom had followed Siva and I on this journey, were the first to learn the good news. It was quite fitting, really, for these are Siva's people, his tribe, and his backbone at work.

I texted a few more people who had shared the journey with us. This was news too good not to share far and wide. And then it struck me. I hadn't shared it with Siva. That made me laugh, and I knew that Siva would understand and laugh, too. Not too long after 5:30 p.m., I called Siva to share the news of the next step in his journey back. I felt the smile down the phone and something else, too. Maybe a little hint of fear? Worry?

The journey back meant that Siva's supervisors could step in and I could step back. He was to change dance partners and learn a new dance step. Siva was to be present at the hospital again, visible in the OR. He would not be unseen, and I would not have to be his torch bearer. He could answer all the questions, and everyone would be able to see and touch their most beloved person.

Now What?

Siva—Recounted May 4, 2019

I once saved someone who probably didn't want to be saved. I was sitting on my aunt's front porch in the village of Kandadevi in India during a welcomed break from medical school, feeling relief from the hustle and bustle. Chatting away, I turned and noticed a man had hung himself from a Banyan tree. As fast as my bare feet would carry me, I ran to the tree with my uncle in hot pursuit. Together, we lifted the man down from the tree. He wasn't breathing, so I used what tools I had and rolled up one of the large leaves from the Banyan tree, inserted it into the man's airway, and breathed life back into him. As the adrenaline wore off, my uncle looked at me and bluntly said, "Now what?" Now what, indeed. As doctors, we pull people back from the edge without always having a plan for their "what's next."

The man I saved turned out to be a vagrant who stayed with us for two days, living in the cowshed. Then he disappeared. I had saved someone and then set him free to who knows what, to hunt out a strong branch on the next Banyan tree?

I would love to work in a village where there are no tools, and you just have to rely on your knowledge and skills. Modern ORs are not like this, of course, with machinery, tools, and people all cluttering the space. Sometimes the chatter can be so loud and too much, and that is when I go quiet. My silence is a cue to others.

Back to the Grind

Siva

Back to the grind wouldn't mean a Monday morning start for me. I was to return on a Tuesday at 8:00 a.m. for the weekly surgical team meeting, very few of which I had missed since the stroke. My three colleagues were to be my supervisors, and I would be the junior. It was quite the change for someone heading for sixty!

The triumvirate had agreed to submit weekly reports on my performance and abilities to the Ontario College of Surgeons. The college's compliance committee had set parameters for us all to follow and complete, so there would be lots of homework and reflection. I had a journal to document the details of every case with which I was involved, and Prema wanted me to start writing in it right away. I left it to one side. Patient demographics are easy to complete, that's why we print out stickers to affix to everything. I was confident, and when I closed my eyes, I was like the bonesetter. I could feel and visualize every step of a surgical procedure; now I just needed to do one. Of course, I had thought long and hard about what it would be like if I couldn't do something. I would be happy to admit that I couldn't and would gladly hand over the reins to one of my supervisors. The most important thing for me was getting back into surgery and getting a licence to practice medicine and perform surgeries independently. For now, I was to have a licence with restrictions; my task was to slowly eliminate the need for those restrictions over the next six to eight months.

A range of surgical procedures would be logged in my journal, and how I carried them out would be documented. Would Siva's "great hands" save the day? My mind said they would, and time would tell like it always did. Of course, being supervised and assisting with procedures carried out by other surgeons meant that I was to be unpaid. I had no right to bill for the work I did. That was the least of my worries, as I had to prove myself capable of being an MRP. The progressive levels of supervision range from high to medium to low. Somewhere along the way, I would attain MRP status. Even when I did, which would afford me the ability to conduct surgery and bill for my time, I had decided not to do so right away. Instead, I allowed my supervisors to bill for their time, since the opportunity cost to them for observing my work versus doing their own was significant; it was a form of karma and payback in a world where time was money.

Fair Is Fair, Purpose of Purpose

Siva

A stroke is devastating. A stroke is an especially devastating thing to happen to someone who relies on the finesse of their brain, hands, and movement. A stroke is devastating for a surgeon, and I will, to this day, never accept that one happened to me. I, who. I, who was invincible. I, who saves lives. I, who am responsible for other people's lives. But I have fought back. My mind's eye had visualized all manner of surgical adventures over those eighteen months. Here I was on the precipice of a return to surgery, and soon I would know how reliable my mind's eye was.

Naturally, I regularly thought about the what ifs. What if it was too much of a grind? What if I didn't have the stamina? What if I couldn't do it? What then?

I remember wondering how would I fill my days if I were no longer a surgeon. A former surgeon and now a retired colleague, had turned to day trading stocks. I'd taken a look and thought that's something I could do. They say you can make $500/day— that would be pretty good pocket money. Prema was skeptical and just nodded her head when I brought it up, as if indulging the whims and dreams of a child.

The daily search online for options led me to a one-year course in regenerative medicine at the University of Toronto. The use of stem cells is undoubtedly the way of the future, so this felt like a good option for a frontier explorer. The hospital, my employer, had suggested options that included managing an e-records transition project. Again, this was the future, but I couldn't even begin to imagine how to manage physician colleagues and encourage them to enter all patient records and monitor online as they happened. I knew how much of a task that would be since they barely have time to get through their morning rounds and scribble down some notes before surgery begins.

It would be far more efficient to pay someone—a nurse, most likely—to enter our data. We are efficient with our time allocation; that's for sure. I can't say that an information technology (IT) project offered much allure or excitement to me. It was a Plan Z, if one at all. In fact, at home we had laughed long and hard about the notion of offering the least technologically savvy surgeon a lead role on an IT project. What a joke.

Knowing that the hospital was looking for ways to use my knowledge and accommodate me was comforting, but it wasn't where my mind was. But an IT project—did they want me out? Did they want me to leave? I was set on returning as a surgeon, so until I could try that and understand how it would be, it was difficult to make any other long-term decisions.

Prema

Siva's search for purpose was very clear and necessary.

From the number of windows open on the computer's browser at the end of the day, it was clear just how curious and searching Siva was. He was searching for a path that would give him purpose. Regenerative medicine seemed like a reasonable compromise, but I worried if even that might have been a step too far at that stage of Siva's career.

Day trading had been thrown up as an option a few times, and my stomach heaved when I thought of Siva spending his days in front of a screen, playing the markets. He belonged in front of a screen, performing endoscopies. If trading was what he ended up doing, then limits would have had to be set. We were not gambling with our financial security.

Siva's brain had been tested to the maximum over those past two years. It had been deprived of oxygen—an area 0.2" across that had been irreparably altered—and then it had been subjected to executive functioning testing that I and my surgeon colleagues had struggled to comprehend or answer. Siva was given the most difficult tests to complete. We joked that he probably would have struggled to complete them before the stroke. But it didn't matter, then; he had nothing to prove, then. In his good-humoured way, Siva joked that "they're trying to make me more intelligent."

A lot of what we focused on and read about post-stroke was loss and deficits. What a person could no longer do. Little is written about how a stroke changes and enhances its victims. Siva's right brain stroke had given him time—time that he had never had before. The stroke had allowed him to spend time with his mother in Malaysia—time that was taken away when he was nine years old. The stroke also enhanced Siva's reactions to funny things, and his laughter is so energetic now that it is infectious. He sees joy in simple things, laughing uproariously at Benji's antics.

Post-stroke, Siva has quite possibly reached enlightenment, allocating his time to the things that matter and finding joy in the simple and mundane.

The Mechanics of Breaching a Frontier

Siva—Recounted June 8, 2019

The CPSO undertaking wanted me to complete fifteen surgeries/endoscopies and by complete, they meant lead. My surgeon colleagues, some of whom I had helped, now saw their role as that of training me and easing me back into surgical life. So, rather than lead surgeries, I was to assist theirs.

I returned to work on Tuesday, June 4, 2019, as planned. As I'd predicted, I was more than ready, so with bags packed, I arrived for our usual 8:00 a.m. surgical team meeting. The welcome was warm, and unlike the past eighteen months, this time I didn't have to go home after the meeting but rather headed to the second floor to the OR for work.

Dressing in my all-too-familiar scrubs brought me back to being Siva. Everything slipped on very easily and right into place, except my cap. The cap sat loosely on my head because I couldn't tie the bow tight enough. I practiced many things, except the simple task of tying a bow. Holding my left arm above my head long enough to cross over the strings was like holding up the weight of the past eighteen months. Eventually, I managed to make a reasonable bow, but nothing close to the fit that I liked. One of the nurses was kind enough to help me re-tie it. As I stood like a child being readied for school, I wondered if I was ready for surgery. Maybe the nurse wondered this too. A surgeon who couldn't tie a bow. What kind of surgeon was that?

Suppressing the doubt, I scrubbed in and entered OR 2. On my first day, I assisted one of the longest-standing surgeons. He made me long standing, too, because I didn't leave work until 6:00 p.m. So much for easing me back into things. He is old school, and his old school mentality meant that he put me through my paces, right from kickoff. So, you want to be a surgeon? Well, then, this is what you must endure. That was the training environment I was raised in, so I knew where he was coming from. Prema was not going to be happy to hear all of this. I thought to myself, dare I tell her?

I assisted with some cases that initially looked simple but turned out to be challenging. Retracting and holding the scope at an unnatural angle with my left hand was a feat of endurance for the first day back and for such a long day. Having expected to assist with a few cases and leave early on day one, I was surprised but certainly not shocked. This is how life had always been for me, how I chose to live my life—pushing, challenging, performing feats of endurance, and breaching new frontiers. I belong in the circus.

When I left at 6:00 p.m., my only thought was "I survived." I think it had become my reaction to everything. I had survived the stroke, the setbacks, the journey, and day one of surgery. I, who.

Prema

I was like a parent who had sent her child off to school for the first time. Really, I wasn't like this when Arjun and Geetha started school. Siva returning to work felt like he was being cut loose and set free, simultaneously. Free to walk the tightrope or swing on the trapeze, with no netting.

I was in the hospital too on Tuesdays, and all day long on that Tuesday, June 4, I wondered how Siva was doing. I called one of the nurses, a friend, and she assured me that all was well. But I needed to hear it from Siva himself. I needed to see how well it was going. I saw him in the surgeon's lounge, chatting happily with his colleagues. We chatted momentarily and in response to my "How is it going?" question, Siva said, "We can chat about it at home." I froze in fear. This must have meant that there had been a problem and that Siva was in trouble. I responded in Tamil, hoping that would afford us the ability to converse privately. Siva just reiterated in English, "Later, at home."

When I finally got my Siva home at 6:00 p.m., I was distraught and angry. They knew this was a man who had been away for nearly two years—a man who had had a stroke. They knew he needed to be eased into things, not committed to feats of endurance on day one. But then it dawned on me that this was how Siva chose to live—on the edge, at the summit, on the frontiers.

The "first day back" euphoria was clear to see. Siva was tired but pleased with how he had endured all that the day had thrown at him. We laughed that he wasn't able to tie a tight enough bow on his cap. What kind of "mother" was I? Knowing that day two would come quickly, I explained to Siva that I had been worried about him all day. I asked him why he was so abrupt in the surgeon's lounge and wouldn't talk to me in our native language. His response was very logical: "Talking in Tamil would just make people think there was an issue." How intuitive, how full of reasoning. Siva's brain was working fine.

Siva

Day two was a good day. I rose early, but I was late leaving the house. I made it to the OR on time, though, picking up speed as I moved through the familiar routines. This day, I was with a younger surgeon, one more in tune with human needs and less driven by old-school endurance. I was relaxed in this environment and when offered the opportunity to suture, I was not exhilarated. The suturing was slower than I would have liked and was a sobering reminder of the journey ahead.

Perspectives—Different Views of the Same Thing

Prema

After one week back on the job, Siva had his first assessment with his colleagues. Siva thought he had passed with flying colours, but the supervisors did not. In his opinion, they were quite harsh; they felt that when he was suturing, he was not using his left hand to pick up skin every time. He argued that it was just a few stitches, and he had done it that way before the stroke. He asked them if they wanted him to be ambidextrous, able to use both the right and left hand well, and they said no. Siva felt that they should have been assessing him in his current state with his disability to see whether, with adaptation, he could perform procedures safely. He thought they were misunderstanding the process and were assessing him like he was a trainee. If they really wanted to assist, they would have helped him adjust and adapt to perform the procedures safely. Wasn't that what the process was all about? Siva knew better than anyone else in the OR how to do those procedures; his cognition was intact, and his body was mostly recovered, but his left limb, which was completely mobile, was not as finessed. It could, however, be trained to adapt. To myself I thought, Siva just needs to adapt.

Though the college intended for Siva to be assessed doing tasks such as scopes and surgery under a high level of supervision, the supervisors wanted him to continue assisting major surgeries for a few more weeks, which was not considered part of the assessment. Siva was crushed. I think that, in his mind, having his colleagues as supervisors meant that they were going to be encouraging and give him more to do, moving things along quickly. He was impatient to move forward because, in his mind, he could do everything.

I advised him to go with the flow; being resistant to the supervisors might lead them to halt the process. The only way he was going to win with them was to keep doing what they asked of him. In his mind, he was doing well. My heart was heavy, so heavy. He was a good man, and he had been through hell and had the courage to do this, but there was a hard journey ahead. I did not know if his colleagues were comparing him to before. There were so many questions that hung in the ether, unanswered and unanswerable.

I spoke my mind to Siva. Perhaps the toll of supervising him was impacting his colleagues too? I reminded him that he was back to being a resident and that there would be no easy journeys. I advised him to bow his head and soldier on. I think Siva realized that he had no choice. Like all things in life, the ice would eventually break, and we would all move on, I hoped.

Siva—June 2019

This whole month passed in anticipation of getting to do more, but except for one supervisor who allowed me to do more, the others just had me assisting. This was not considered in my assessment, so I had nothing to report to the college, as there had been no supervision of me performing any procedure.

They thought that they were acclimatizing me to surgery again. They did not realize that I had been practicing this in my head for the last eighteen months. There were good days and not-so-good days; it was an emotional rollercoaster.

Prema had me watch a motivational talk by Brené Brown in which she talked about courage and vulnerability. She essentially said that it takes courage to show one's vulnerability. My spirit soared hearing her as I felt vulnerable in a task and process that I had no control over. I made a commitment to myself to keep persevering.

Siva—July 6, 2019

The return to work—the pursuit of a licence—is far more challenging than any of us ever envisaged. My colleagues, who were now my supervisors, were different. Maybe they were behaving differently—protecting their reputations—or maybe I just saw them differently. They were my colleagues, so it was difficult to have them pick over my work. I didn't use my left hand to suture, they would tell me during our weekly assessment meeting. I have always favoured my right hand, so had they scrutinized me closely before the stroke, they would have known that I had never really used my left hand, at least not to the extent that they thought I should be.

There I lived, under a microscope, and some days—many days—I wished it was under a rock. I, who.

I was not the only one who was frustrated. It seemed that I frustrated my evaluators. I tried to keep my head down and get on with all that they had asked of me. That would have been endurable if I had felt that they were trying to help me progress. But they were not. They were slow in allowing me to lead surgeries; in fact, they were not allowing me to lead any. So, I had not yet fulfilled any part of my undertaking with the college.

If I didn't lead, then I couldn't lead. Instead, I was being led—led to the beat of someone else's drum.

Under a high level of supervision, attending weekly meetings that pointed out life-long patterns, habits, and foibles—these are the conditions under which I now operated.

Except that I didn't operate. I watched and helped at the margins. In the OR, I was on the margins. I sensed that I was not wanted there, an unwelcome presence. Pressure built, but I held my tongue. The pressure continued to build. This journey to the centre of my existence was difficult and frustrating. Why? Because I was not in control of the journey, and I hadn't surrendered to the process. I was trying to steer the boat when someone else had their hand on the tiller. Mental power, the will to succeed, the desire to breach new frontiers—these traits were all still there, but some days I couldn't help but feel that they were waning.

I was not a junior surgeon or a trainee; I was an older man whose brain and body had been changed by a stroke, and my role as a surgeon was being diminished and downplayed. My role had been to serve as a reminder to all other surgeons and doctors that life can change in the blink of an eye, in the smallest blockage of an artery in the brain. Like all things, though, the lesson and reminder I served up to people were short-lived, and very quickly, people re-entered their own rat race and forgot about how life can change in an instant.

Wherever He Goes, Ego Goes Too

Prema—July 2019

The path to enlightenment means that the ego must go. Siva was not on this path. His ego, built on who he once was, the surgeon he once was, was dominating and driving him. He was like a spoiled child: refusing to converse with or confront his supervisors. Hiding. Looking for excuses and alternatives.

I understood how difficult it had been for him. I empathized with his journey and all that he had faced and still continued to face. But at the centre of Siva's world was Siva. Not me, his wife. Not his two children. In fact, we were being cast away. Oh, how that hurt to say out loud. After twenty-six years of marriage, it looked as though "I, who" never became "we, who."

In the face of adversity, Siva was running and capitulating. His latest plan was to go live in India to train the next generation of surgeons in the small town where he once lived. I laughed at the innocence of this dream. He didn't seem to realize that India was not waiting for him to save the world. The India of his childhood and early training was gone. The rules and regulations would still exist, and the journey would not be any easier. Siva thought it would be because he would be happy there; his family would be around. But we were his family. We were here in Canada. We were being discarded.

I was all out of the fight. I had nothing left to give. Of course, Siva would use that as a reason to leave, citing it as me being unable to take care of him and give him what he needed. Let him go to India, let him find another wife, I thought.

Single-handedly, I had managed everything because Siva always put work and himself first. I knew that I could survive; I had been the sole caretaker of our home, our children, and our marriage for years. To be relieved of one of these would be a bonus for me.

Was I angry? Yes. Sad? Extremely. Tired? Very. So, I was surrendering to whatever plan had been put in place for me by being more supreme than Siva.

Every Tuesday was stressful. My heart broke, seeing my husband reduced to a bundle of nerves, because judgment was going to be made at the morning meeting. He did not feel like he was being supported to make progress. He felt judged, and his progress was not determined by his performance but rather more by his supervisors' timelines. I prayed so hard every day, so God could get him through this by giving him strength and confidence. Why did he need to go through this, after all that he had already endured?

We were at a phase in life when most people in Siva's situation would have retired. So, Siva having chosen to go through it was on him, and he would have to endure it. We were not receiving much empathy for what he was enduring! Everyone around thought he was fortunate to even be given the opportunity. But in his mind, he could do this, and he was not allowed to progress like he wanted. He was being put through the wringer. I could feel what he was going through. Cognitively he was sound. His knowledge was unimpaired and with rehabilitation his left hand, the non-dominant hand, is functioning but weaker than before so in his mind he can go back to doing what he did before with some compensation and adaptation. He was frustrated that his supervisors were expecting him to perform the way he would before his stroke. They were not able to assist in supervising him as he was now, post-stroke.

The pressures mounted and when they did, they had to be released somehow and somewhere. On July 25, 2019, our house was the scene of an explosion, with a meltdown and family meeting. It was interesting to witness my husband listen to his children more than to his wife; it means that we have been married a long time!

He felt belittled and demeaned and that he was being treated worse than a resident. This caused some distancing and alienation from his colleagues, and he was straying into tantrum territory. I told Siva to give it all up, as I could not handle the stress anymore. Hearing Arjun and Geetha talking to him was fascinating. They sounded so sensible, so grown up.

We realized that Siva was now at ground zero.

Siva

India is where I feel happy. With my family around me, I always feel safe and connected. Here in Canada, I was not connected, and I was nobody now that I was no longer a surgeon of stature. So, the ties and pulls of a happy childhood and a desire to return to halcyon days were dominating my thoughts. Thoughts that should really have been focused on work.

"Appa, are you leaving us?" my daughter asked. Even that question didn't shake me, leading me to think that my brain had truly been altered. I knew that I would never leave her, but I also felt that she no longer needed me. She was at university now, studying to be a doctor. She didn't need me, I thought. My needs were paramount.

Was I being selfish?

Yes, I was, but until I was happy, I would not stop.

Regrouping for the Final Ascent

Siva

After a stressful and uncertain return to work, I looked forward to our summer vacation in Yellowknife, Northwest Territories, in early August. Our last family vacation had been more than twelve months previously. It was an amazing two weeks. I came back rejuvenated, reenergized, and ready to return to the assessments with my supervisors, with vigor.

But the rug was pulled from under my feet.

My supervisors stated that they did not feel comfortable assessing me due to my disability, or in their words, my "different body biomechanics." They recommended to the CPSO that my assessment needed to be done in a tertiary centre (one associated with a university, a teaching hospital), with individuals used to training residents.

I was crushed and felt like I had been betrayed and that they had wanted me to fail all along. The final trap door opening under me was my supervisor's refusal to continue the process until I was able to make arrangements with the university. They did, however, agree to complete the minor surgery supervision. For that, I was grateful.

I accepted my predicament and persevered in minor surgeries for two months, keeping up with chart reviews. I met with colleagues at the tertiary centre at University of Western Ontario (UWO) and they agreed to assess me. A mini fellowship was designed for this process. I was and have continued to be, very grateful.

There was another two-month delay to starting this mini fellowship, but during this time, I found that I really enjoyed performing minor surgeries, and my practice got busier than ever. I even started contemplating that it could be my entire practice. I thought I could accept it. I still had a purpose for getting up in the morning, seeing patients, doing skin excisions, and reconstructing them beautifully, then following up with patients to see the final outcome—a full circle treatment. I absolutely could do this.

But I was Siva, and I breached frontiers, so I planned to see how the rest of the mini-fellowship process went, no stress. I could accept whatever the final outcome was.

On December 12, I heard from the CPSO: I was deemed independent to perform minor surgeries. Hallelujah!

The Battle Within

Siva

With the holiday season and the end of a decade approaching, I looked forward to downtime with family. But for my spirit to soar, I needed to have gratitude, forgiveness, and love in my heart. I had to let go of the bitterness that was consuming me. I was bitter about my current predicament, my body that did not perform like my mind wanted it to, my uncertain future, and not knowing what my purpose was.

To attain true freedom, I needed to be able to observe problems instead of becoming lost in them. I was grateful for how much I had recovered through my psyche, while the world kept focusing on what I had not attained: the full and free movement of my body and my endurance. If possible, I wanted my full licence to have the freedom to volunteer on medical missions or work in remote communities. I wanted the freedom to choose where and how I would work.

My assessment schedule with the surgeons in London was set. My plan was to go with the flow for the next six months to find out how much I could do. I planned to take it one day at a time and let life unfold without trying to control it.

I worked with different surgeons at the university. They were very supportive. The challenges I faced were trying to perform colonoscopies using the technique currently taught, and I was not allowed to do it the way I had always performed colonoscopies. I appreciated learning a new technique but trying to do this in my recovering state made me look and feel like a novice. I also began to develop an increasing left shoulder pain with any abduction or rotational shoulder movements. This became increasingly worse when I was performing an endoscopy. I did not share this information with my supervisors as I felt it would appear that I was not up to the task.

I kept up with my assessments and it culminated one day while doing a scope with a severe, searing pain in my left shoulder, so severe that I had to pass the scope to my supervisor and excuse myself. I was later diagnosed with a rupture of the long tendon of my left biceps. After the rupture, my shoulder felt better, but I had a bulge in my left biceps, like Popeye! My orthopedic colleagues advised me that it would be best to manage this conservatively. I took a break to allow my shoulder to heal but could never restart the assessment as the COVID-19 pandemic then put a halt to everything.

I was supervised for two months and concurrently managed to do minor surgeries and completed over three months of chart reviews, finally getting to a place where I was now certified *Independent to do Minor Surgeries*. This was an achievement compared to being unable to stand two years prior. There was so much more to accomplish over the next six months and beyond—there were more frontiers to breach.

I was continuing with my minor surgery practice and was enjoying it immensely. I was beginning to feel grateful . . .

Global Pandemic

Siva

The chief of surgery position at my hospital was posted, and as usual, none of my surgical colleagues were interested in taking it up. I was the last to even consider this but compared to my colleagues who were working full time, I did have more time. So, on the premise that I would be helping the surgical program and with encouragement from Prema, I applied. I went through the interview process and was offered the position in February 2020.

I thought that this would be a good opportunity to develop my leadership skills. I was not very good at checking my emails regularly, and all that had to change. I was determined to try. The pandemic was announced in March 2020, and within six weeks of holding this position, I was suddenly dealing with an unprecedented situation, with a flurry of activity, meetings, OR closures, and changing guidelines, all while doing my best to keep up on how to follow the public health guidelines. Having to deal with lots of meetings, disgruntled surgeons, and anxious staff was quite challenging for me, as I did not have the opportunity to grow into and learn the role. What I realized was that when one is struggling, a few people lift you up. It is usually the same people, my friends, but there is always someone to bring you down. They also tend to be the same people. These colleagues did not feel that I was able to manage the role, so I stepped down graciously in October 2020. I was ascending Everest and got thrust down to the Mariana Trench. My stress level, however, fell immediately. The only person who was unhappy that I had taken on this role was my mother, who was concerned that I was inviting more stress into my life. Mothers always know best.

The pandemic roared on. Resident training became challenging, and my situation was not a priority for the university. So, I had to wait.

God has a way of presenting things when He thinks you are ready. A suggestion from a colleague stating that my endoscopy skills could also be assessed by a gastroenterologist made me seek out my colleague in my hospital, who agreed to supervise me. CPSO was notified, and the usual undertaking and my assessment in endoscopy started and went splendidly.

I was certified to perform minor surgeries and endoscopy independently in June 2022.

Epilogue

Prema

Now, Siva is busy. He works almost every day of the week, and he is tired at the end of the day. He is filling his schedule but reminds himself frequently not to overload his plate.

I am so proud of his accomplishments and that he has come so far. To me, I think that everything he is doing is enough for him. He is doing scopes, minor surgeries, and helping people with the routine and daily things that need to be done but without the stress of doing calls or very complicated cases. I would be very happy for him to continue with this regimen, but he is stubborn and wants to continue fighting for his full licence. He is fighting for his freedom.

Freedom for Siva is being able to take two weeks off when he pleases to complete a mission with a volunteer program abroad, such as Doctors Without Borders. Siva would work as a surgeon in a remote community somewhere. Other possibilities have crossed his mind, such as wanting to go to Northern Canada to act as a locum.

However, he cannot do any of these "free" possibilities because he does not have his full licence. To Siva, this means that he is still facing his frontier.

I don't know what his future holds, but in my heart, he has accomplished so much, and this is more than good enough for me. Siva enjoys his downtime and rest. Even after the time that has passed, he is still recovering from a neurological injury. Patients get tired, so I fear that if he has his full practice back, he may not cope well with the stress.

Knowing my Siva, I know that these are decisions that only he can make. However, as we continue to move forward, now on the other side of the mountain, they are decisions that he includes me in, asking for my advice and sharing the journey as equals.

Siva and I have become a strong team, enduring great climbs and suffering tough falls. We have learned the power of providing each other with strength and support when the other needs it the most. Working on this book has provided us with a therapeutic release of the anger, confusion, frustration, sadness, and fear that controlled our lives over the better half of these past five years. While I wish to this day that the stroke hadn't happened to our Siva, I am grateful for where our family is today and for how strong we are together.

We cannot change the past; we can only move forward. Each day may bring new challenges, but it may also bring new possibilities.

I know that Siva's journey is far from over. I can see the twinkle in his eye as he continues to push for his ultimate freedom as he continues to push through new frontiers.

This time, I feel confident that whatever new frontier life places in front of our climb, we will pull each other up, ascending together.

Siva

Receiving my certification to perform minor surgeries and endoscopy independently in June 2022 was just the news I needed to hear; however, this is only the beginning of the next phase of my journey.

I will not stop until I have reached my freedom, until I have my full licence again. This is a new frontier, one that I will endure great challenges to get through.

I have to find a surgeon locally to supervise me. Unfortunately for me, all of the current surgeons are too young, so I have to wait longer. Waiting is not a new concept for me after the years I have endured. But this time, waiting continues to push me further and further away from having been able to operate on major surgeries. I am still operating, and my schedule is full, keeping me busy with the minor surgeries that I perform four times a week. These are not considered major surgeries, so I fear there will be problems from the college about them.

All this has been difficult to wrap my head around. I have done this for so long pre-stroke, but now, I have not done this for too long. Will I still know how to do it?

I know in my heart that I am capable. I want to complete this journey, to conquer this frontier, because only with a full licence can I feel that I have freedom, that I have not lost. In my retirement, I had dreamed of participating in voluntary work abroad and doing locums; this is how I have always looked at myself in my future years. While I am proud of how far I have come, I am Siva, and I am not ready to quit.

While I continue to face some of these internal struggles, as there are always frustrations, I am better able to cope with them. It's simple: just take deep breaths.

It has helped to work regularly in ambulatory care, an environment in the hospital that feels like a family. I enjoy going to work every day. I am happy that I am able to go to work and be with people who welcome me, encourage me, and care for me. They are my family, my home away from home. When we have long weekends and I cherish the time with my wife and children when they are home, though I miss the work; however, when I am at work, I sometimes gripe that there is too much work. I understand that this comes with the work. As Prema says, I can be quite stubborn.

All in all, frustrations are fewer, I am happier and my family at home as well as in ambulatory care have become my happy places.

I accept the fact that we will always be on a journey. I acknowledge the fact that I am in a much better place now than I was, as I am able to do so much more for myself and keep myself busy. I no longer just sit at home staring at the walls, wondering what I am going to do with the rest of my life. Achieving my certification for minor surgeries and endoscopy provided me with work again which gives me fulfillment.

It also provided me with a new family in ambulatory care. This has taught me that people are a part of my fulfillment.

They look out for me, and it is something that I am grateful for after the many disappointments and struggles that I have faced with both people and situations over the past few years.

I am in a newly found happy place where I am able to see many patients and remove many skin cancers. I get to see the fruits of my labour every day when I follow up with those patients. This gives me a lot of fulfillment and pride that I have made it back this far.

However, I cannot see myself doing this for another fifteen years.

I long for my own freedom. I want to do things on my own terms. After having been pulled and prodded through the process of regaining my certification, I have witnessed what it feels like to be tethered to something where you do not really have autonomy.

If I have learned anything from this journey, it is that even if all the doors seem to be closed, just wait. Be patient. One will open.

I will continue to make my next move.

I don't know what the next stage of this climb holds. I do know that I will continue to fight. I will continue to push through my frontier.

I am Siva. I am a stroke survivor. My next climb is only just beginning.

Thoughts on the Regulatory and Life Expedition

Siva

My hope for this book is to help anyone going through a stroke journey, one that may even mirror the one I have gone through. Here are some facts and insights:

- In a second, your life can change forever.
- I have heard repeatedly that every stroke is different, every person is different—this is true. My journey will not be anyone else's, but I hope that my insights and experiences will help someone else in their time of need.
- Persevering and trying to return to your previous self is a lot of hard work, and you need a burning desire to recover. A good support network is vital. Mine was primarily my wife and family.
- If you are a post-stroke surgeon and want to return to practice, it will be your Everest. There are no protocols

in place to help surgeons return to work. You need to get representation with CMPA (who are excellent), and it is much easier to communicate with the CPSO through them than it would be as an individual. I am hoping my journey has created a precedence for other post-stoke surgeons.

- The CPSO needs to be assured of your competence and ability to practice safely as they are protecting the public, not you.

- The Royal College of Surgeons certifies you as a surgeon and does not get involved in the return-to-work process; they do not have any resources laid out to help a surgeon return to practice.

- You are fighting alone and must rely on your surgeon colleagues to help you with the process. Remember, they will also be quite stressed by the many legalities laid out by the CPSO.

- You must really want to do this, as you will stand alone in the spotlight and have to face many judgments and critiques.

- As a surgeon trying to get back to surgery post-stroke, I see now that it would be far easier to change career paths to teaching or management. It would be easier still to retire.

- I would be remiss not to mention that you need a person like Prema in your life and on your side. She is the scaffold upon which I have climbed and built my life; she is my rock.

Prema

As the caregiver of a stroke patient, here is what I now know to be true:

- When your spouse has a stroke, you have a stroke together.
- Preceding this event, I lived my life very optimistically, furnished with positive thoughts and inspiration. I think this has made me stronger and that the universe has long prepared me for this stroke journey.
- When I was in the process of recovery with Siva, I just focused on the moments and dealt with what needed to be done while along the way planning for the next steps, so he had all the necessary therapy to recover. There are so many steps, and it is an easier journey if the stroke patient is a willing participant. Siva generally was, but we of course faced our challenges.
- I was lucky to have my career so that financially, we were stable and could fund all of Siva's needs. To also be in a financial crisis during an experience like this would be very difficult, not to mention extremely stressful.
- Physical recovery is much easier and more measurable than psychological recovery.
- Returning to work for a post-stroke surgeon is an achievement but brings its own challenges. Confidence or its lack thereof is stressful. Having a life coach helps.
- There will be periods of doubt throughout the journey. All you can do is be a support and allow your stroke partner to figure out what their next steps are. Siva

picked the road less travelled with all its challenges. There were many dark days of self-doubt and wondering if he should quit. He would jokingly say that the stroke was the easy part!

- Building my strength and stamina was essential to our journey; I found that music helped a lot, prayer, and a few good friends. I also started painting and discovered that I had a latent talent. Painting is very relaxing.

- The support you will initially receive from colleagues and friends is overwhelming and touching in the beginning. When you are two years out and the journey is ongoing, you feel much more alone, as, understandably, everyone gets busy with their own lives. The few people still reaching out to you are true angels, and you will forever cherish them because they help you get on with your life and through your day.

- Sometimes, the people you expect the most from disappoint you the greatest. It is best not to place too high expectations on any one person or group.

- Writing this book started off with the aim of it becoming a resource to help people going through a similar journey, but we found that talking to our ghost writer was very therapeutic too.

- We have to realize just like all kinds of discrimination like racism, sexism, ableism is also present in our society.

- Ableism is the discrimination of and social prejudice against people with disabilities based on the belief that typical abilities are superior. At its heart, ableism is rooted in the assumption that disabled people require 'fixing' and defines people by their disability. Like racism and sexism, ableism classifies entire groups of people as "less than" and includes harmful stereotypes, misconceptions, and generalizations of people with disabilities. (quoted by Ashley Eisenmenger, Disability inclusion training specialist in Access living)

- It may sound like a cliché, but everything happens for a reason—and this pause we have had in our life has given us so much more perspective on what is important and the true nature of people. It has set a course for how we will live the rest of our lives.

Abbreviations used in book

CPSO-College of surgeons and Physicians of Ontario
CMPA-Canadian Medical protective agency
RCPSC-Royal College of Physicians and surgeons
MRP-Most responsible physician
tPA-Tissue Plasminogen activator
OR-Operating room
ER -Emergency room

Resources—Signs of Stroke

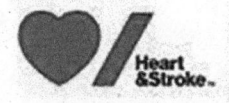

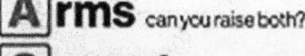

Face is it drooping?
Arms can you raise both?
Speech is it slurred or jumbled?
Time to call 9-1-1 right away.

Heart &Stroke™

Local Chatham-Kent Protocol for Stroke

The Chatham-Kent Health Alliance (CKHA) is having good success in treating suspected strokes with two new policies.

When the patient arrives . . . the doctor will perform a very quick assessment of the patient to confirm that they are having what appears to be a stroke and the patient immediately goes for their CT.

The images from the CT are then sent to a neurologist at the London Health Sciences Centre. When the patient returns to the emergency department, staff wheel a screen to the patient's bedside for the Telestroke portion of the new practice.

The physician from London will be able to see the patient while looking through the CT images and will recommend treatment for the patient's stroke.

Click here to read the full *Chatham Daily News* article by Tom Morrison, "New Policies Mean Faster Treatment for Stroke Patients".

Chatham Kent Health Alliance has also introduced a Code Stroke announced over our hospital speaker system to alert all the members of the stroke team, so the incoming patient receives timely care.

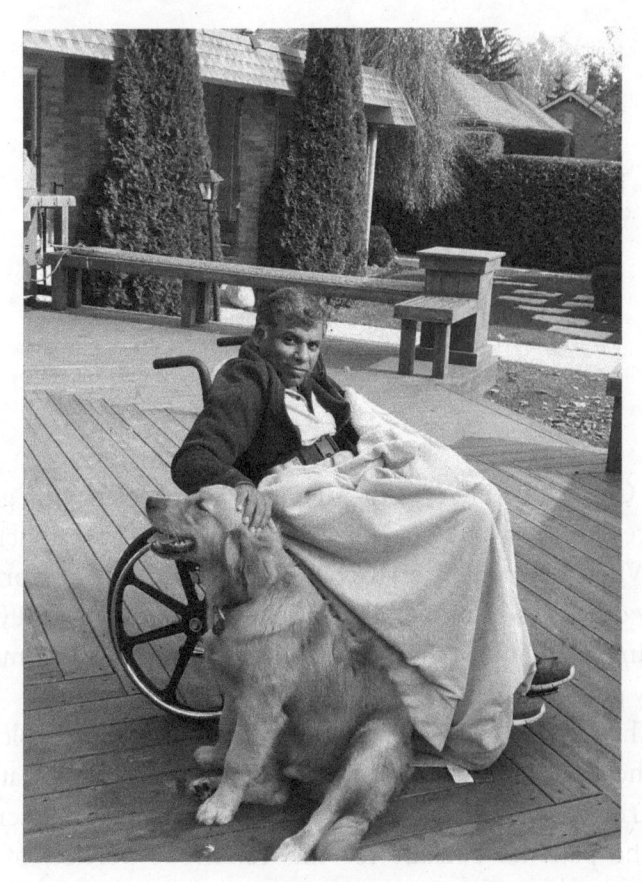

1 month after stroke

Printed in Canada